Sawsan Daoud
Nouha Farhat
Mariem Damak

Idiopathic generalized epilepsy in adults

Sawsan Daoud
Nouha Farhat
Mariem Damak

Idiopathic generalized epilepsy in adults

ScienciaScripts

This book is a translation from the original published under ISBN 978-620-6-70398-3.

Publisher:
Sciencia Scripts
is a trademark of
Dodo Books Indian Ocean Ltd. and OmniScriptum S.R.L publishing group

120 High Road, East Finchley, London, N2 9ED, United Kingdom
Str. Armeneasca 28/1, office 1, Chisinau MD-2012, Republic of Moldova, Europe
Printed at: see last page
ISBN: 978-620-7-13021-4

IDIOPATHIC GENERALIZED EPILEPSY IN ADULTS
DAOUD SAWSAN, FARHAT NOUHA, DAMAK MARIEM, MHIRI
CHOKRI NEUROLOGY DEPARTMENT
CHU HABIB BOURGUIBA, SFAX, TUNISIA

INTRODUCTION

Epilepsy is characterised by a cerebral predisposition to generate epileptic seizures (ES)(1).idiopathic epilepsies (IE), which are the focus of this study, comprise a group of syndromes defined by specific clinical and electroencephalographic features(2).The pathogenesis of this form of epilepsy is not fully understood. It has been suggested that the term "idiopathic" should be deleted from the nomenclature of the epilepsy classification, since it signifies the absence of a known or suspected aetiology other than a possible hereditary predisposition (3). It is therefore more meaningful to refer to this group of syndromes as genetic epilepsies. However, it is rare for the genetic mutation(s) causing a patient's epilepsy to have been determined. The experts at the International League Against Epilepsy therefore decided that the term idiopathic generalised epilepsy would be acceptable specifically for the group of four epilepsy syndromes: childhood absence epilepsy, juvenile absence epilepsy, juvenile myoclonic epilepsy, and epilepsy with isolated tonic-clonic generalised seizures (2).These epilepsy syndromes represent approximately 20% of all epilepsies, but less than 1% of epilepsy research (4). This imbalance reflects a lack of awareness of the diagnostic difficulties that clinicians may face and of the real impact of these epilepsies on patients' quality of life. In fact, new data show that patients with IE may go undiagnosed, especially in cases of late onset or drug resistance. Focal epilepsy may also be misdiagnosed in these patients if there are focal electroencephalographic abnormalities or asymmetric seizures. All these difficulties in diagnosing and managing idiopathic generalised epilepsy could be resolved by epidemiological studies aimed at defining the clinical characteristics of these epileptic syndromes and understanding the overlap and differences between them. In our study, we analysed the demographic, clinical and electrical characteristics of idiopathic generalised epilepsy syndromes in an adult Tunisian population, in order to determine the characteristics of IE in adults and to look for distinctive features between these IE syndromes.

The objectives of our work were to :

• Estimating the frequency of AEs compared with other types of epilepsy in adults

• Describe the main epidemiological, clinical and electroencephalographic features of the various AR syndromes.

• Classify our patients according to the latest classification of epileptic syndromes (2).

• Evaluating the response to antiepileptic drugs (AE) and the evolution of these epileptic syndromes

• Try to find distinctive features between the different syndromes EI

PATIENTS AND METHODS

1 TYPE OF STUDY :

We conducted a retrospective study in the neurology department of CHU Habib Bourguiba Sfax including patients who consulted or were hospitalised for epilepsy over a 5-year period (2019-2023). Patients were contacted to collect missing data.

2 STUDY MATERIALS :

2.1 Inclusion criteria :

Our study included :

• Patients over the age of 18 who consulted our department between 2019 and 2023 for epilepsy (either newly discovered, or as part of the follow-up of their illness, or referred to us from other health facilities for further treatment).

• Patients meeting the definition of epilepsy as proposed by

ILAE in 2014 (1).

• Patients with a diagnosis of AE according to the classification of epileptic syndromes published in 2022 (2).

2.2 Exclusion criteria

We excluded patients with :

• Symptomatic epilepsy or epilepsy of unknown cause

• Late-onset generalised epilepsy (onset after the age of 30)(5) with no family history of epilepsy, for which cerebral magnetic resonance imaging (MRI) has not been performed.

• Genetic focal epilepsies (autosomal dominant nocturnal   frontal epilepsy and familial temporal lobe epilepsy).

• Recurrent acute symptomatic crises (metabolic, withdrawal, etc.)drugs...)

3 STUDY METHODS

3.1 Collection of data

We drew up a study form for collecting anamnestic, clinical and para-clinical data on all patients. We specified the following parameters for each patient:

3.1.1 Anamnestic data :

We have specified :

–Epidemiological data :

Age, sex, geographical origin, marital status, level of education, profession, age at first consultation, marital status, social security cover.
–The existence of any parental consanguinity

–Family history: medical, surgical, epilepsy and psychiatric illnesses
–Personal history: perinatal circumstances, history of febrile seizures, cranial trauma, central nervous system injury, general or psychiatric illness, etc.
–The history of the epilepsy: age of onset, time to consultation, type of seizures, frequency and timing of seizures, presence of contributing factors, nature of treatment and response to treatment.

3.1.2 Neurological examination :

–Examination of higher functions.

–Looking for focal neurological signs :

• Pyramidal syndrome

• An extrapyramidal syndrome

- Cerebellar syndrome

- Cranial nerve damage

3.1.3 Examination

3.1.4 The results of para-clinical investigations :

3.1.4.1 Critical and/or inter-critical electroencephalogram)

The electroencephalogram (EEG) was performed using a bipolar set-up with a 10/20 system of 21 electrodes, lasting a minimum of 20 minutes with intermittent light stimulation (SLI) and two hyperventilation tests (HPN) lasting at least 3 minutes. We analysed the background rhythm, paroxysmal EEG abnormalities and the response to the various provocation tests (HPN, SLI). This examination was performed in the neurophysiological exploration unit of the Sfax neurology department. For patients who had had several electroencephalograms, we considered the data from the pathological tracing.

3.1.4.2 Morphological brain imaging:

Cerebral MRI and/or CT scans were performed in all patients included in our study.

3.2 Input and analysis of data

The various data were entered using Microsoft Office Excel 2010 and analysed using SPSS 20 software.

- Quantitative variables were expressed as the mean $\pm$ one standard deviation and qualitative variables as a percentage or headcount.
- For all statistical tests, the significance level (p) was set at 0.05.

- We used the Chi 2 test to compare percentages.

- We used the Student(t) test to compare the means

1 SUMMARY RESULTS

1.1 Prevalence :

We collected 407 records of patients with epilepsy. We included 127 cases of idiopathic epilepsy. The incidence of AE was 31.2% of all patients with epilepsy. We classified our patients according to the age of onset of the epilepsy. F o r electro-clinical syndromes in children, three patients had EAE. For electro-clinical syndromes in adolescents and adults, 100 patients presented with EI-CGTC, 22 patients were followed for EMJ and only 2 patients presented with EAJ (**Figure 1**).

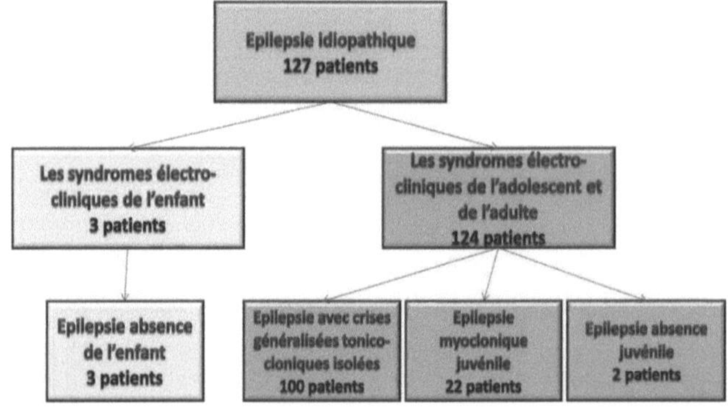

Figure 1: Distribution of patients according to electro-clinical syndromes

1.2 demographic data

1.2.1 Gender

There was a slight male predominance, with a sex ratio of 1.15 (Figure 2).

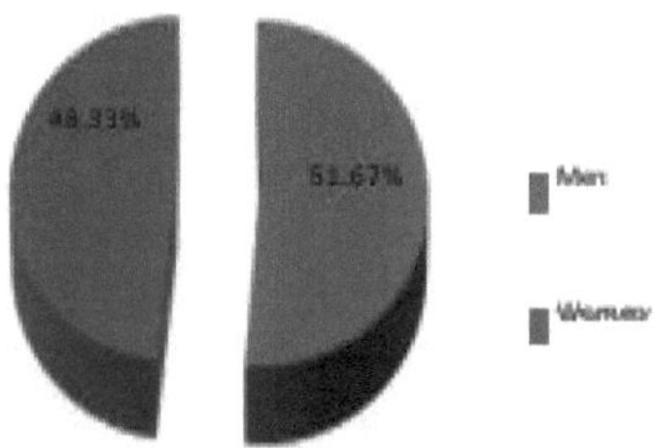

Figure 2: Breakdown of patients by gender

1.2.2 Educational level and professional

The distribution of educational levels among all patients was as follows Follows (Figure 3):

• Illiterate and primary level: 55.11

• Secondary and higher education: 44.89

At the time of the study, 59.85% of patients were not enrolled in school and were not receiving any education. not professionally active (Figure 4).

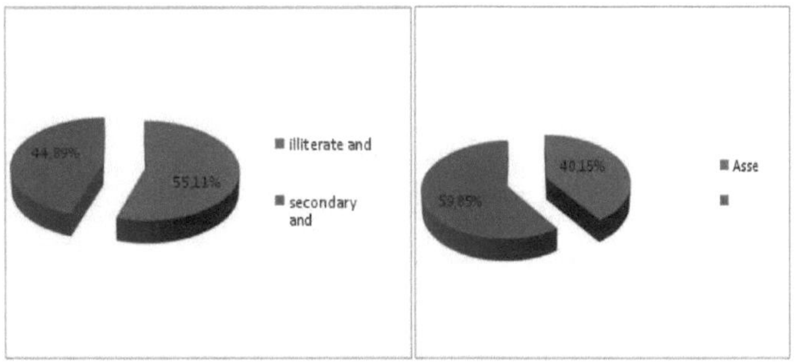

Figure 3: Distribution of patients by level of education

Figure 4: Breakdown of patients by professional status

1.2.3 Marital status

Of our patients, 49.6% were single, 45.66% married, 1.5% divorced and 3.14% widowed (Figure 5).

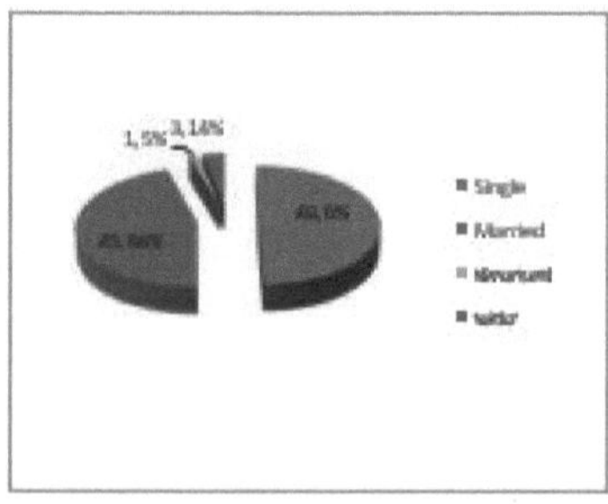

Figure 5: Breakdown of patients by marital status

1.3 Genealogical data :
1.3.1 Origin geographical

Our patients came from various governorates in southern Tunisia. They were of rural origin in 51.18% of cases.

1.3.2 Consanguinity

Parental consanguinity was found in 38.58% of cases (Figure 6).

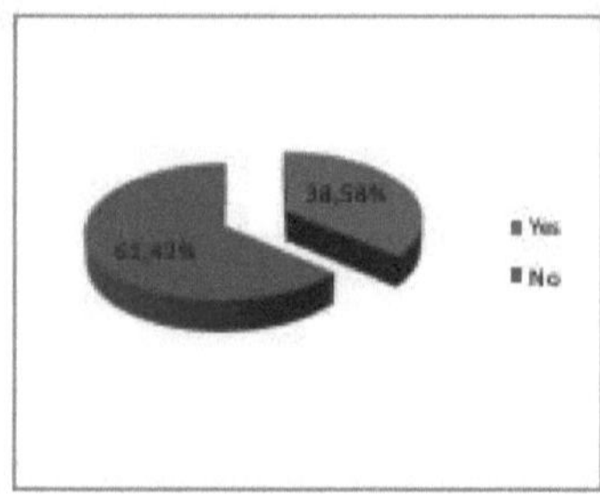

Figure 6: Distribution of patients according to consanguinity

1.4 Clinical data :

1.4.1 History of febrile seizures(FC) :

A history of CF was found in 19.68% of patients (Figure 7).

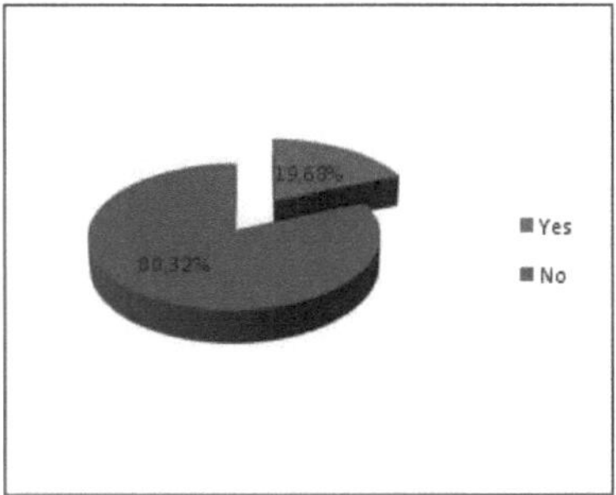

Figure 7: Distribution of patients according to history of febrile seizures

1.4.2 Family history of epilepsy :

The family survey identified a family history of epilepsy in 31.49% of patients (Figure 8).

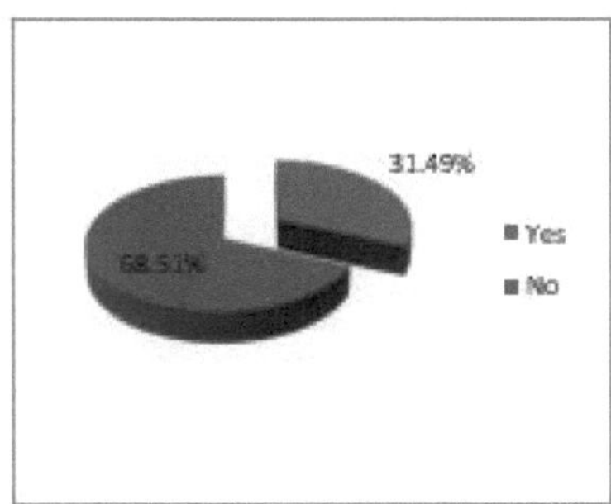

Figure 8: Distribution of patients according to family history of epilepsy

1.4.3 Age of onset of epilepsy

The mean age of onset of epilepsy was 17.83 ± 9.8 years, with extremes ranging from 1 to 49 years and a peak between 11 and 20 years (Figure 9).

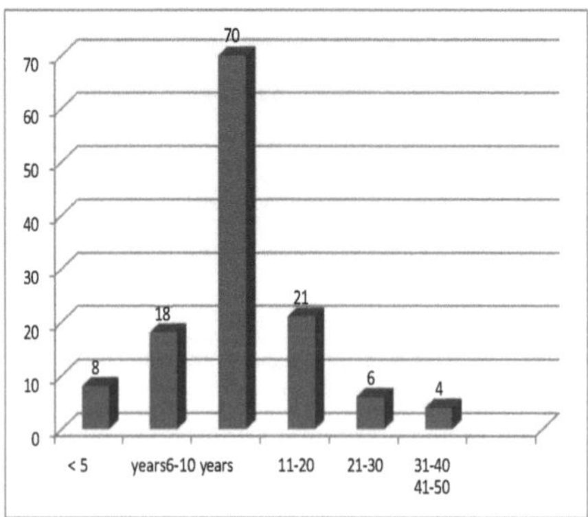

Figure 9: Distribution of patients by age of onset of epilepsy

1.4.4 Progression time of epilepsy

The mean duration of epilepsy was 15.65 ± 8.22 years, with extremes ranging from 1 to 40 years.

1.5 Electroencephalogram :

EEG was performed in 116 patients. Intercritical abnormalities were recorded in 41.38% of cases.

1.6 Brain imaging :

All our patients underwent cerebral CT and cerebral MRI. performed in 46 patients. Imaging was normal in all cases.

1.7 Antiepileptic treatment :

1.7.1 Number of anti-epileptic treatments :

At the time of the study, 62.2% of patients were on monotherapy. Dual therapy was required in 30.7% of patients, while the addition of a third AE was ecessary in the remainder (Figure 10).

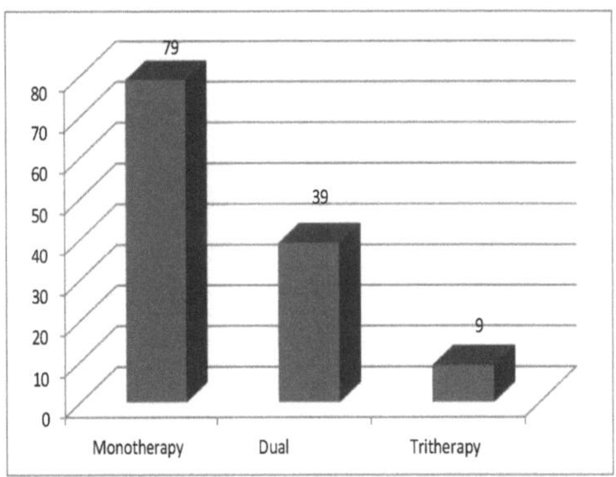

Figure 10: Breakdown of patients by number of antiepileptic treatments

1.7.2 Response to treatment antiepileptic

Progression was favourable in the majority of patients, since the epilepsy was pharmacologically sensitive in 88.19% of cases.

2 RESULTS ANALYTICAL

2.1 Electro-clinical syndromes in children :
2.1.1 Epilepsy absence of the child

Three of our patients were being monitored for EAE (Table I).

Table I: Epidemiological, clinical, electrical, therapeutic and evolutionary characteristics in the childhood absence epilepsy group

		Patient 1	Patient 2	Patients 3
Gender		Woman	Men	Men
Consanguinity		Yes	No	No
Age		20	22	19
F history of epilepsy		Yes (Figure 11)	Yes	No
CF history		No	Yes	No
Age at start (years)		4	3	7
Type of absence crisis		Typical simple	Typical simple	Typical simple
Other types of crisis		No	CTCG	CTCG
E E G	Background rhythm	Normal	Normal	Normal
	Anomaly inter reviews	No	Puffs of OP at 3Hz (Figure 12)	No
	Location		General	
	SLI	No effect	Photo-training	Photo-response paroxysmal: generalised PO
	HPN	Physiological slowdown	Generalized OP discharge (Figure13)	Physiological slowdown
Treatment		VPA	VPA	VPA+PB
Evolution		Pharma-sensitive	Pharma-sensitive	Seizure if a contributing factor (lack of sleep, exposure to unlight, etc.).sun)
EME		No	No	No
Trauma		No	No	Yes

ATCDF: family history; CF: febrile seizure; CTCG: generalised tonic clonic seizure; SLI: intermittent light stimulation; HPN: hyperpnoea; PO: peak wave; VPA: sodium valproate; PB: phenobarbital; EME/Status epilepticus.

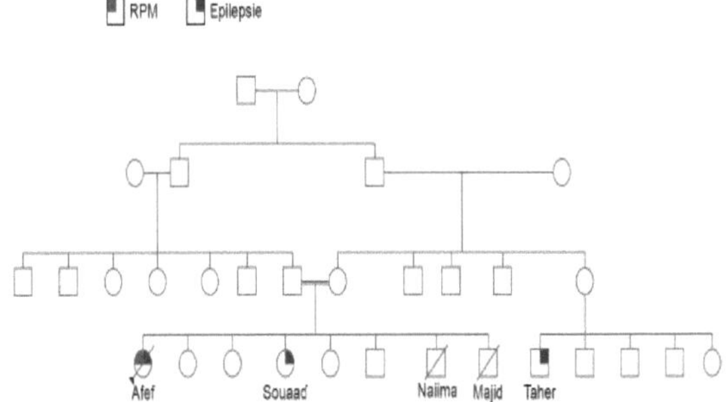

Figure 11:Patient 1's family tree

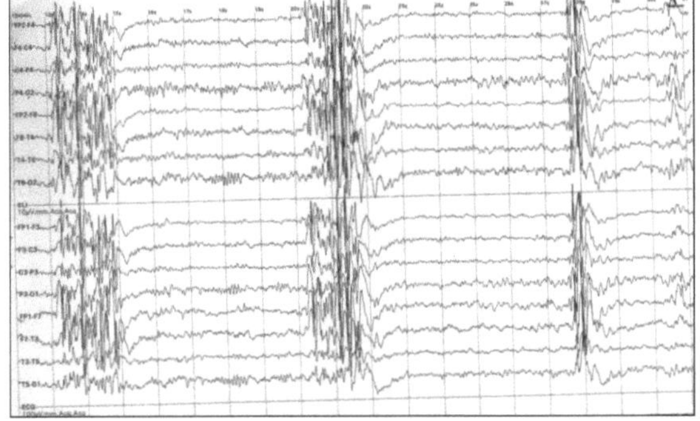

Figure 12: An inter-critical EEG of patient 2: generalised OP puffs

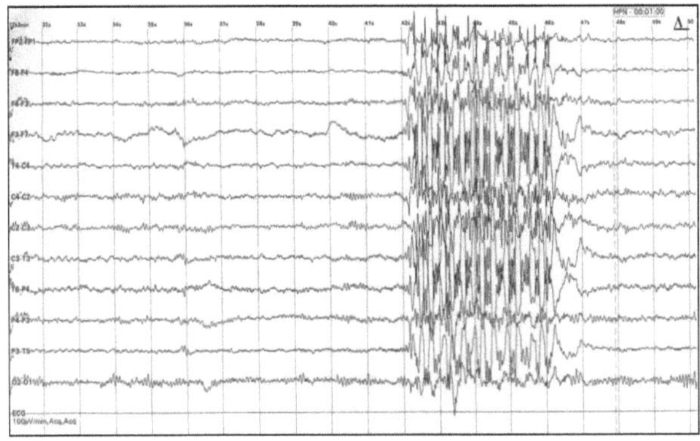

Figure 13: An inter-critical EEG of patient 2 showing generalised OP

discharge triggered by HPN

2.2 Electro-clinical syndromes in adolescents and adults:

2.2.1 Idiopathic epilepsy with isolated generalised tonic-clonic seizures (EI-CGTC):

In 100 patients, we retained the diagnosis of AE-CGTC (i.e. 24.57% of all epileptics and 78.7% of AEs).

2.2.1.1 Gender :

There was a predominance of males, with a sex ratio of 1.27 (Figure 14).

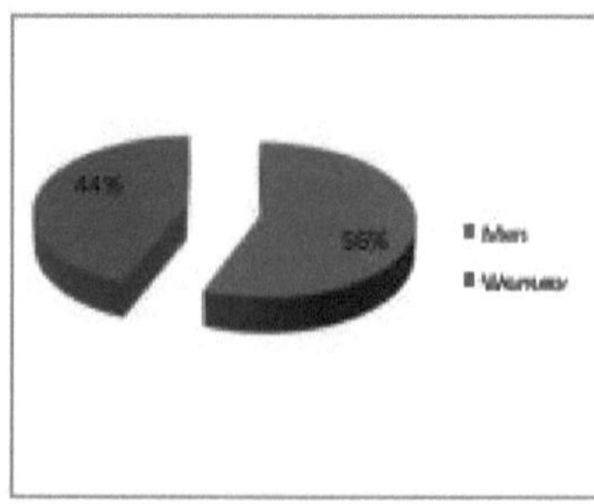

Figure 14: Gender distribution of patients in the isolated tonic-clonic seizures group

2.2.1.2 Consanguinity :

Parental consanguinity was found in 40% of patients (Figure 15).

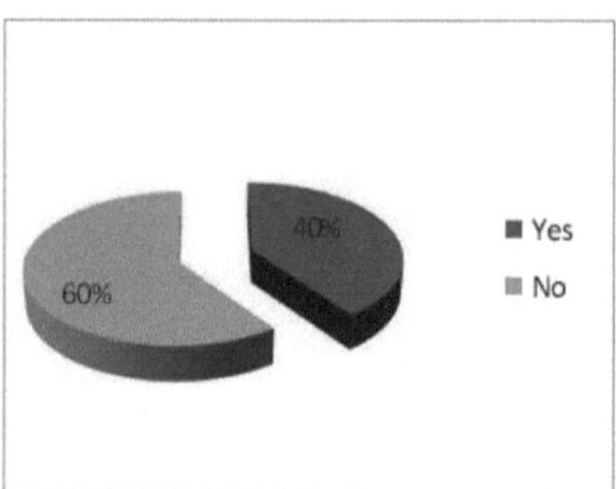

Figure 15: Distribution of patients in the epilepsy group with isolated tonic-clonic generalised seizures according to consanguinity

2.2.1.3 History of febrile seizures :

A history of CF was noted in 20% of patients (Figure 16).

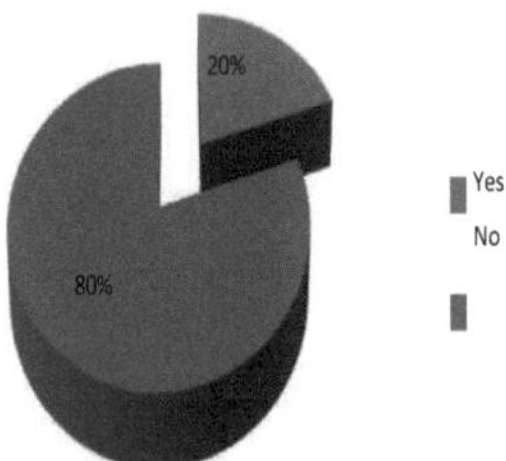

Figure 16: Distribution of patients in the epilepsy group with isolated tonic-clonic generalised seizures according to history of febrile seizures

2.2.1.4 Family history of epilepsy: The family survey found a family history of epilepsy in 29% of patients (Figure 17).

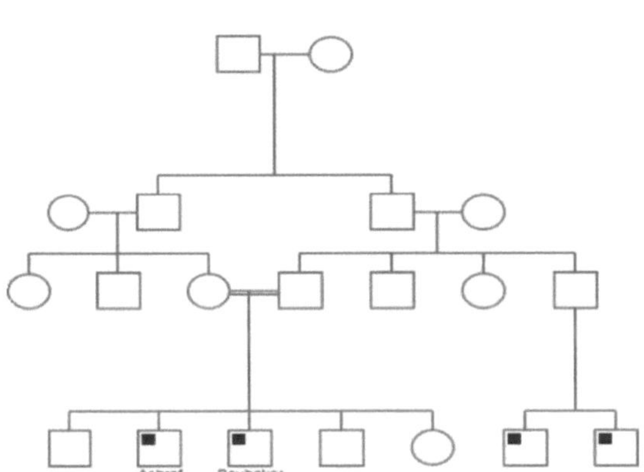

Figure 17: Family tree for idiopathic epilepsy with isolated tonic-clonic generalised seizures

2.2.1.5 Age at onset :

The mean age of onset of epilepsy was 18 ± 10.24 years, with extremes ranging from 1 to 49 years and a peak between 10 and 19 years (Figure 18).

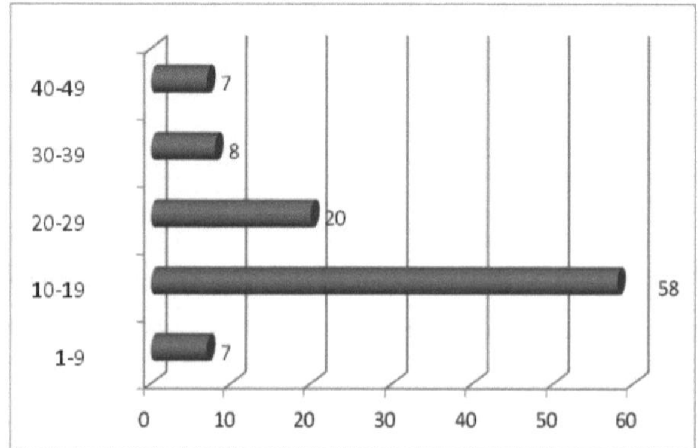

Figure 18: Distribution of patients in the epilepsy group with isolated tonic-clonic generalised seizures according to age of onset of epilepsy

2.2.1.6 Seizure schedule :

Seizures occurred at different times for different patients (Figure 19).

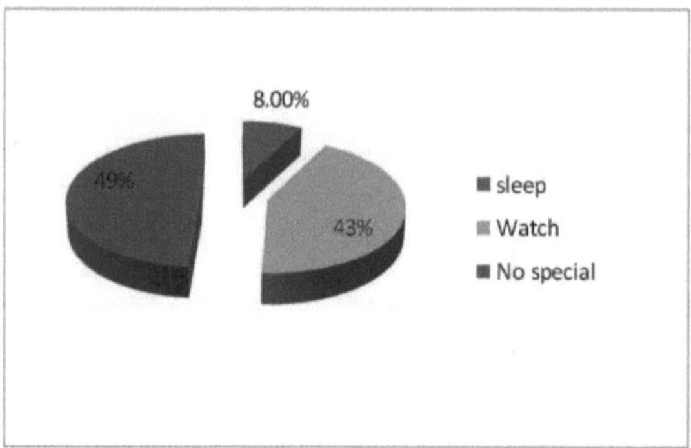

Figure 19: Distribution of patients in the epilepsy group with isolated tonic-clonic generalised seizures according to seizure schedule

2.2.1.7 Clinical photosensitivity :

Clinical photosensitivity was noted in only 2% of patients.

2.2.1.8 EEG :

EEG was performed in 90 patients. A critical EEG was recorded in 3 patients. The background rhythm was normal in 85 patients. The EEG was without abnormality in 68.8% of cases, and in the remaining cases intercritical paroxysmal abnormalities were recorded. Spikes (P), peak waves (PO) and slow waves (OL) were the most frequent abnormalities (Figure 20). An anterior predominance of generalised abnormalities was noted in two patients (2.22% of all recordings) and inter-critical focal abnormalities were present in 13.3% of EEGs (frontal and temporal in 10% and 3.3% of cases respectively). In the remaining cases, the inter-critical anomalies were generalized (Figure 21). 5.55% of patients showed photosensitivity to the EEG (Figure 22). Activation of hyperpnea abnormalities (HPN) was found in 4.44% of patients (Figure 23).

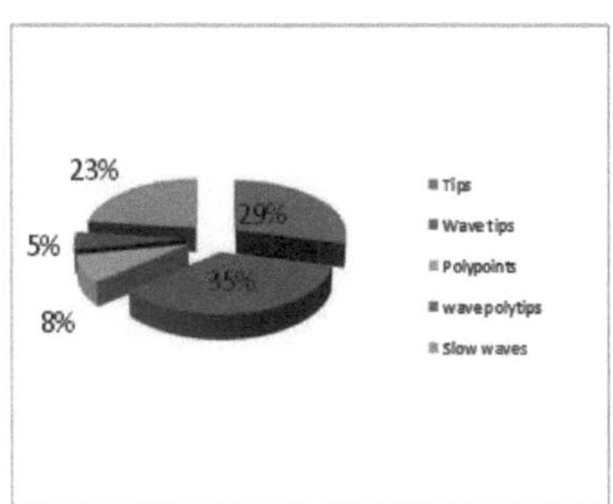

Figure 20: Types of EEG abnormalities observed in the group with isolated generalised tonic-clonic seizures.

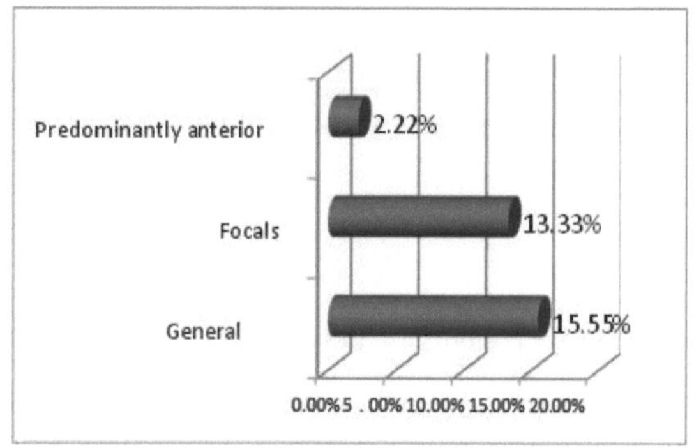

Figure 21: Topography of electrical anomalies in the group of patients with epilepsy with isolated tonic-clonic generalised seizures

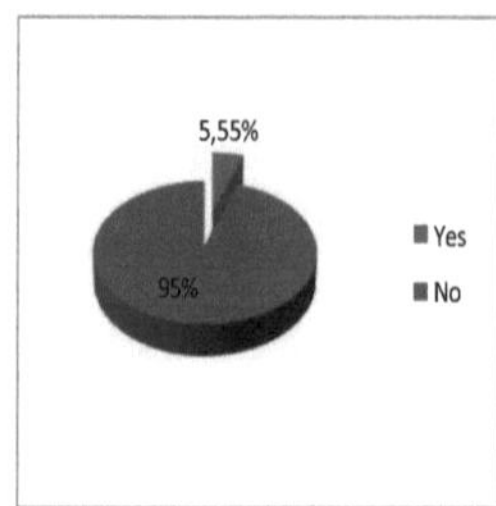

Figure 22: EEG photosensitivity in the isolated tonic-clonic generalised seizure epilepsy group

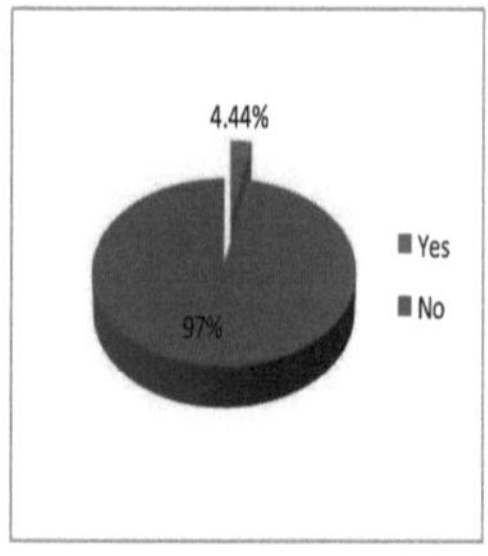

Figure 23: Activation of abnormalities by hyperpnoea in the epilepsy group with isolated tonic-clonic generalised seizures

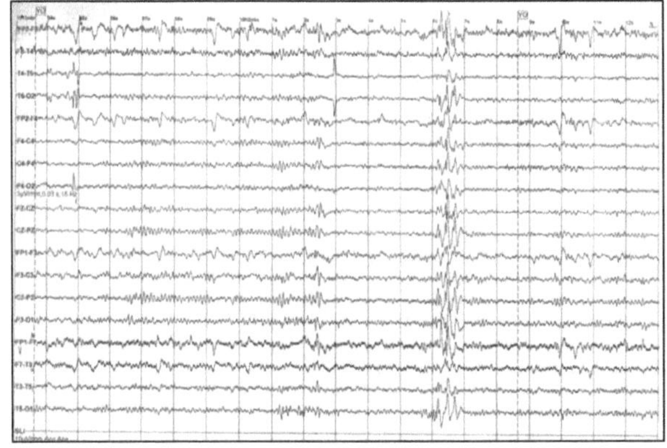

Figure 24: Example of EEG abnormalities in the epilepsy group with isolated tonic-clonic generalised seizures showing generalised PO and PPO flares.

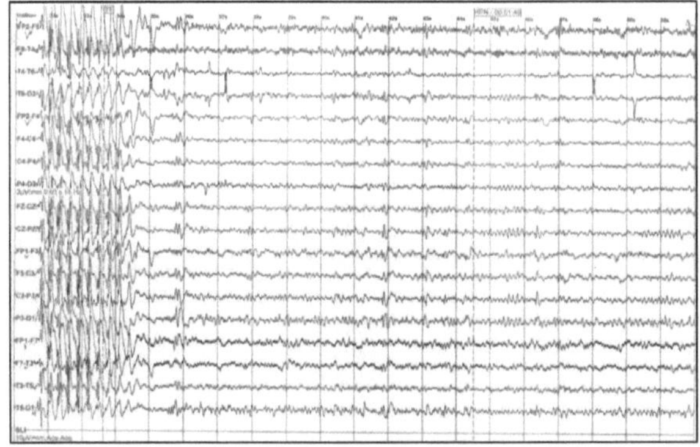

Figure 25: EEG in the epilepsy group with isolated tonic-clonic generalised seizures showing activation of generalised spike-wave discharges by hyperpnoea.

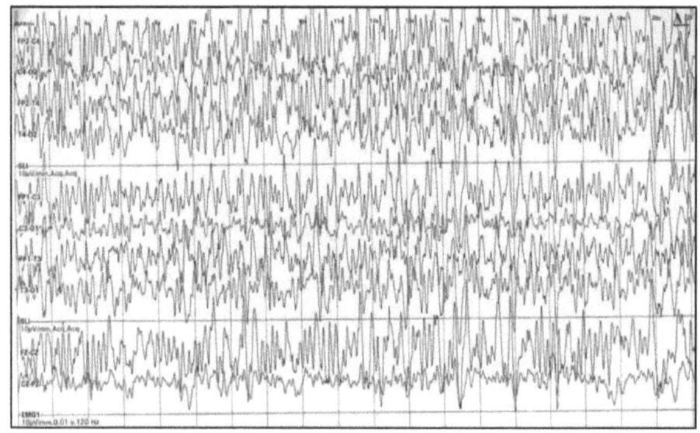

Figure 26: A critical EEG in the isolated tonic-clonic generalised seizure epilepsy group showing a discharge of generalised poly-spikes.

2.2.1.9 Anti-epileptic treatment:

All patients were treated with AE. At the time of the study, 58% of patients were on monotherapy, 33% on dual therapy and 9% on polytherapy (Figure 27). Sodium valproate (VPA) was the most common drug used in the study. prescribed, followed by carbamazepine (CBZ) and phenobarbital (PB) (Figure 28).

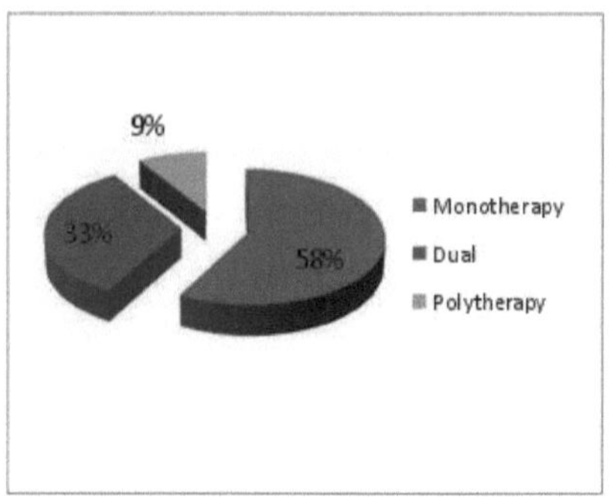

Figure 27: Number of antiepileptic treatments in the group with isolated generalised tonic-clonic seizures

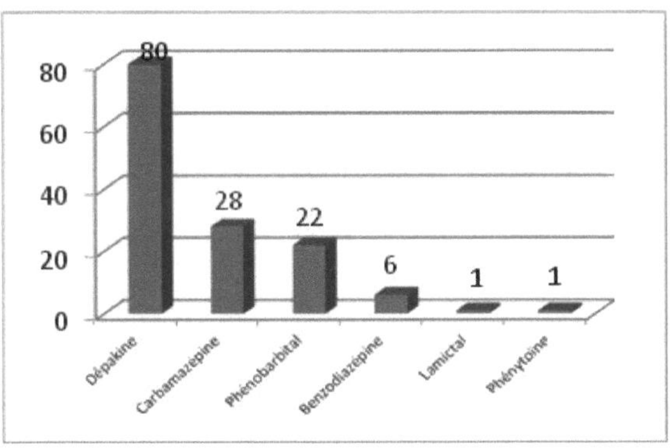

Figure 28: Antiepileptic treatment prescribed for epilepsy with isolated generalised tonic-clonic seizures

2.2.1.10 Evolution of crises:

Epilepsy was pharmacosensitive in 85% of patients, while 15% showed drug resistance. The use of polytherapy was justified in 9 patients, while in the remaining patients, the addition of a third AE treatment was avoided because of intolerance (allergy, impotence, hepatic cytolysis, tremor, somnolence, etc.). Critical trauma and status epilepticus occurred in 20% of patients each.

2.2.2 Juvenile myoclonic epilepsy (JME) :

Twenty-two patients were being treated for epilepsy in the context of a JME.

(17.32% of idiopathic epilepsies).

2.2.2.1 Gender :

Women predominated, with a sex ratio of 0.69 (Figure 29).

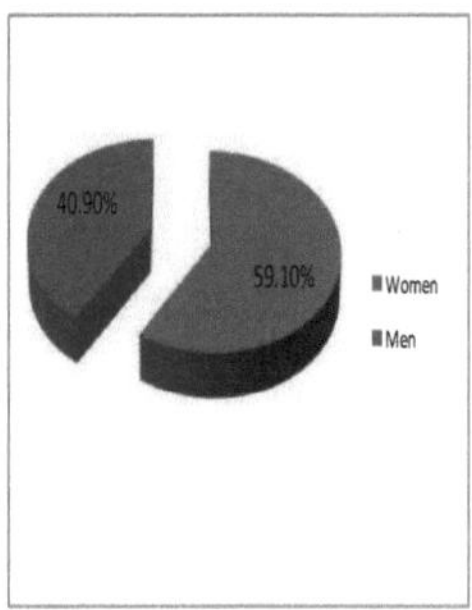

Figure 29: Gender distribution of patients in the juvenile myoclonic epilepsy group

2.2.2.2 Consanguinity :

Parental consanguinity was found in 31.8% of patients (Figure 30).

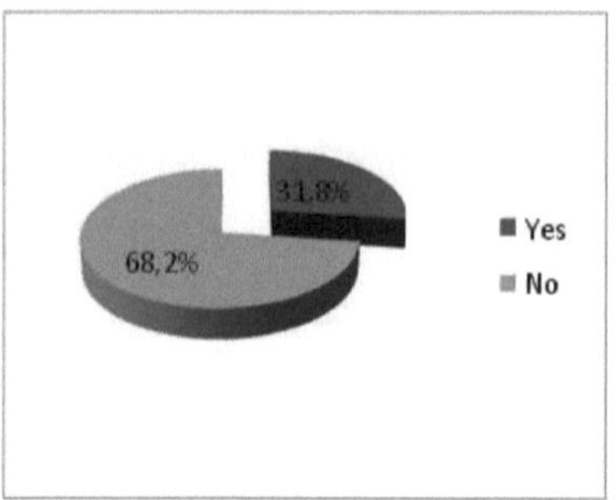

Figure 30: Distribution of patients in the juvenile myoclonic epilepsy group according to consanguinity

2.2.2.3 History of febrile seizures :

A history of CF was found in 13.6% of patients (Figure 31).

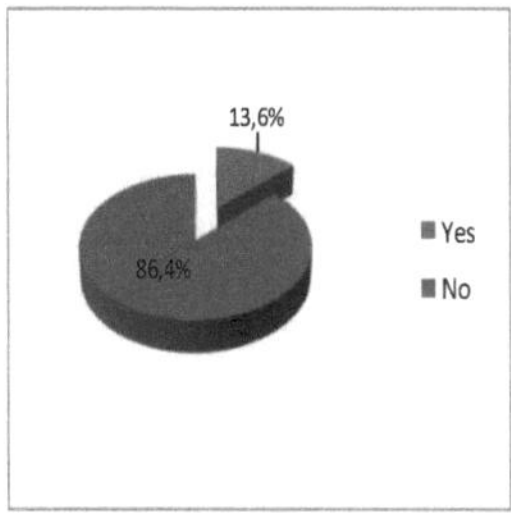

Figure 31: Distribution of patients in the juvenile myoclonic epilepsy group according to history of febrile seizures

2.2.2.4 Family history of epilepsy: The family survey found a family history of epilepsy in 40.9% of cases (Figure 32, Figure 33).

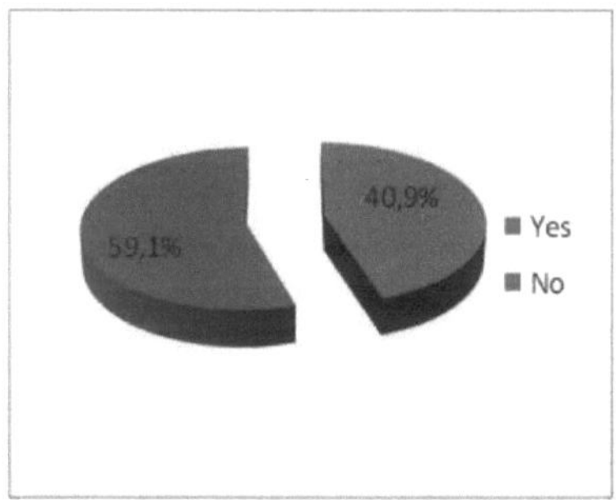

Figure 32: Distribution of patients in the juvenile myoclonic epilepsy group according to family history of epilepsy

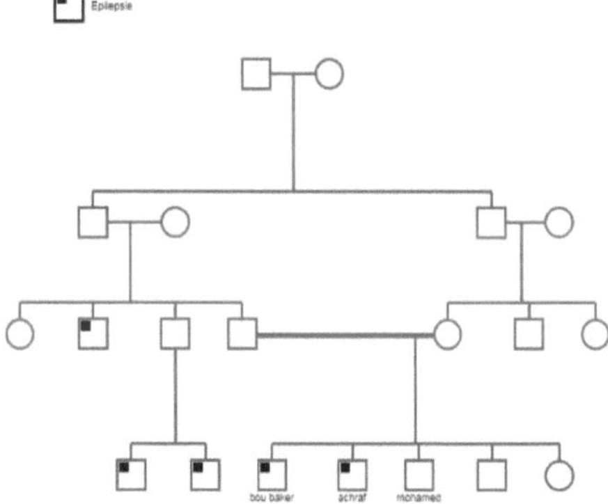

Figure 33: Family tree of a patient treated for juvenile myoclonic epilepsy

2.2.2.5 Age at onset :

The mean age of onset of epilepsy was 18 ± 7.43 years, with extremes ranging from 8 to 32 years, and a peak between 12 and 18 years (54.54% of patients).

2.2.2.6 Clinical features of seizures :

▶ Inaugural seizures:

In our series, upper limb myoclonus was the first type of seizure in 9 patients (40.9% of cases). Generalised tonic-clonic seizures (GTCS) initiated the seizures alone (8 patients: 36.36%) or associated with myoclonus in 4 patients (18.18%). The absence of seizures was the first sign in only one patient (Figure 34).

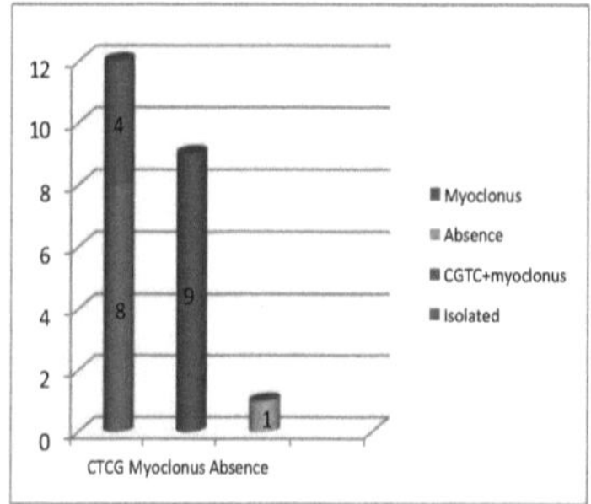

Figure 34: Distribution of patients in the juvenile myoclonic epilepsy group according to inaugural seizure symptomology

▶ Type of seizures during evolution:

Focal myoclonic and CGTC seizures were present in all patients. Absence seizures were also present in 27.27% of patients, and focal seizures were observed in only one patient (tonic motor focal seizure) (Table II).

Table II: Distribution of patients in the juvenile myoclonic epilepsy group according to seizure symptomatology during the course of the epilepsy.

Type of crisis	Percentage
Tonic-clonic generalised seizures	100%
Focal myoclonic seizures	100%
Absences	27,27%
Tonic focal seizures	4,54%

▶ Seizure schedule:

Seizures occurred in the morning on waking (generalised myoclonic-tonic-clonic seizures or CGTCs, or upper limb myoclonus) in 41% of patients (Figure 35).

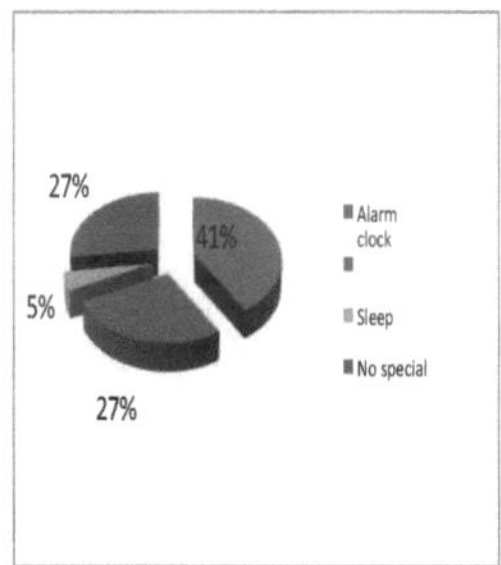

Figure 35: Distribution of patients in the juvenile myoclonic epilepsy group according to seizure schedule

▶ Clinical photosensitivity:

Clinical photosensitivity was present in 22.7% of patients.

2.2.2.7 EEG :

EEG was performed in 21 patients. The background rhythm was normal in all cases. The tracing was normal in 28.6% of patients, while it showed intercritical paroxysmal abnormalities in the remaining cases. Isolated PO and PO discharge were the most common abnormalities (57.14%). PPO was observed in 19.04%

of patients, while PP was only recorded in 4.7% of patients (Figure 36). The abnormalities were generalised in the majority of cases (61.9% of all EEGs), while an anterior predominance of discharges was noted in 2 patients. Focal abnormalities associated with generalised abnormalities were recorded in 2 patients (Figure 37). EEG photosensitivity was present in 23.8% of patients (Figure 38, Figure 39). Activation of hyperpnoea anomalies was noted in 33% of patients (Figure 40). Photoentrainment was recorded in 3 patients (Figure 41).

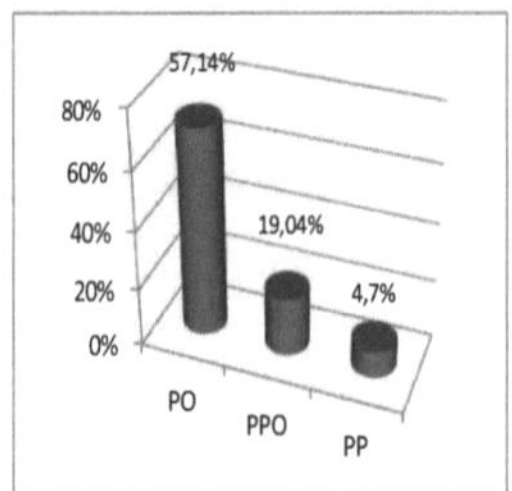

Figure 36: Types of EEG abnormalities in the juvenile myoclonic epilepsy group

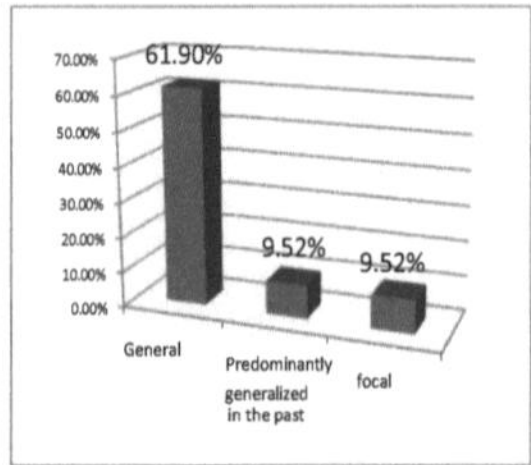

Figure 37: Topographies of electrical abnormalities in the juvenile myoclonic epilepsy group

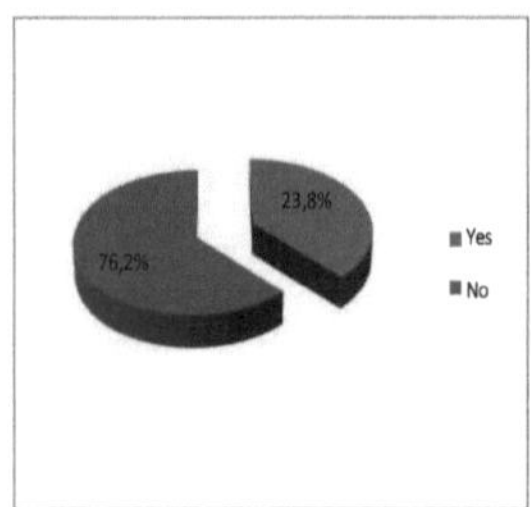

Figure 38: EEG photosensitivity in the juvenile myoclonic epilepsy group

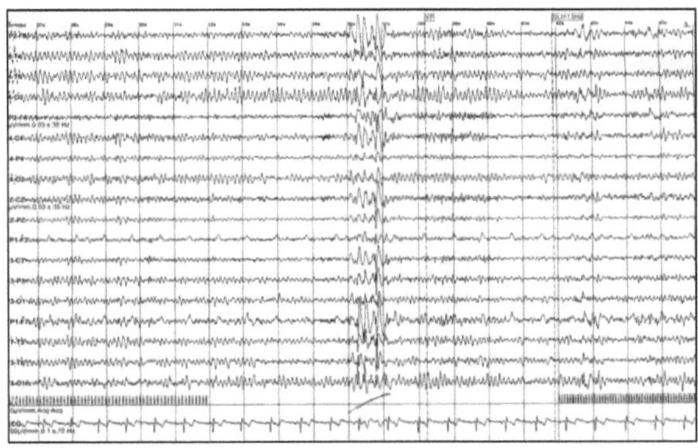

Figure 39: An EEG in the juvenile myoclonic epilepsy group showing a flush of OP triggered by intermittent light stimulation.

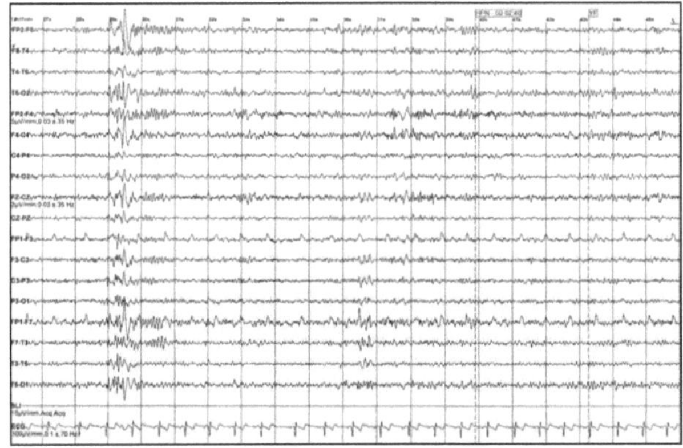

Figure 40: An EEG in the juvenile myoclonic epilepsy group showing PPO generalised, predominantly anterior, triggered by hyperpnoea

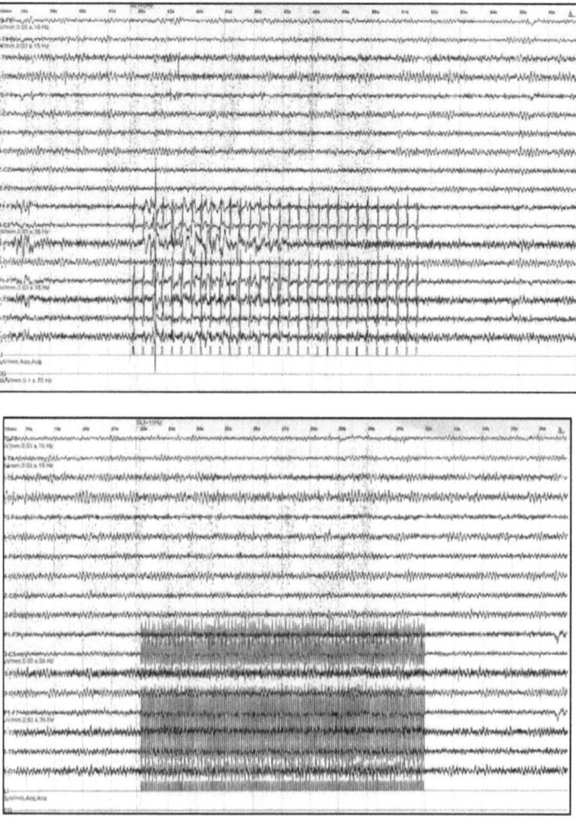

Figure 41: An EEG in the juvenile myoclonic epilepsy group showing photo-training

2.2.2.8 Anti-epileptic treatment:

All patients received antiepileptic treatment. VPA was the most commonly prescribed drug, followed by lamotrigine (LMG), levetiracetam (LEV), PB and benzodiazepine (BZD) (Figure 42). At the time of the study, the majority of patients were on monotherapy, while the use of dual therapy was more common. required for 4 patients (VPA+LMG, CBZ+LEV, VPA+BZD, VPA+PB) (Figure 43). LMG was prescribed at a dose of 100 mg/day for our 2 patients.

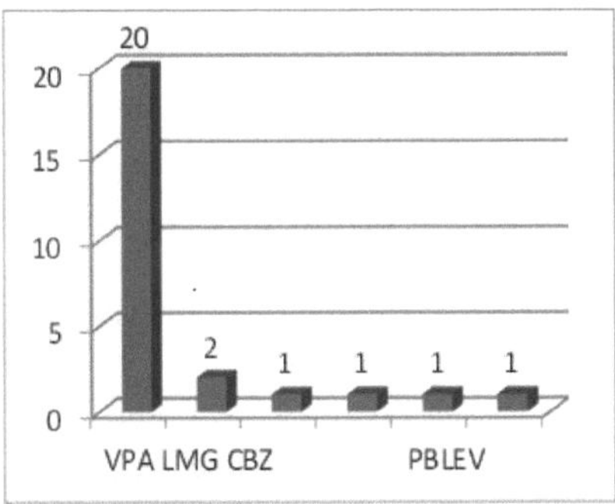

Figure 42: Anti-epileptic treatment in the juvenile myoclonic epilepsy group

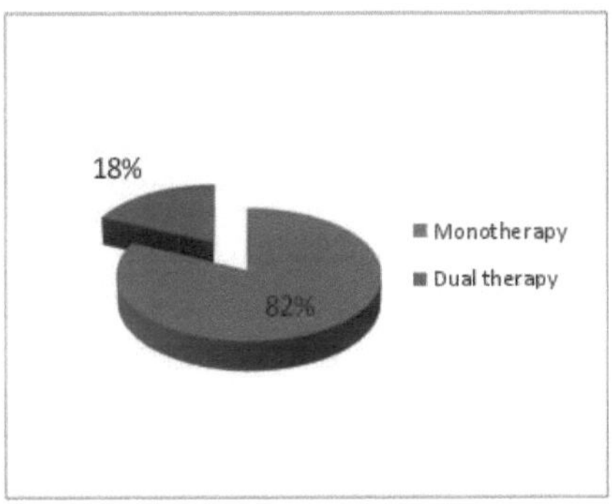

Figure 43: Number of antiepileptic treatments in the juvenile myoclonic epilepsy group

2.2.2.9 Evolution of crises:

Epilepsy was pharmaco-sensitive in all cases. Only one patient had critical trauma and one had status epilepticus.

2.2.3 Epilepsy absence from :

Two patients were being followed for juvenile absence epilepsy (Table III).

Table III: Epidemiological, clinical, electrical, therapeutic and evolutionary characteristics of patients in the juvenile absence epilepsy group

		Patient 1	Patient 2
Gender		Woman	Men
Consanguinity		No	Yes
Age		22	20
F history of epilepsy		No	No
CF history		No	Yes
Age at start (years)		20	19
Absence		Typical simple	Typical complex
Other types of crisis		No	CTCG
E E G	Background rhythm	Normal	Normal
	Inter-critical anomalies	Wave point	Wave point
	Location	Predominantly anterior	Predominantly anterior
	SLI	No effect	No effect
	HPN	Physiological slowdown	Physiological slowdown
Critical EEG		Yes	No
Treatment		LEV	VPA+BZD
Evolution		Pharma-sensitive	Persistence of some seizures
EME		No	Yes
Trauma		No	Yes

ATCDF: family history; CF: febrile seizure; CTCG: generalised tonic clonic seizure; SLI: intermittent light stimulation; HPN: hyperpnoea; LEV: levetiracetam; VPA: sodium valproate; BZD: benzodiazepine; EME: status epilepticus.

2.3 Statistical analysis :

We compared the clinical characteristics and the electrical abnormalities observed in EI-CGTC and EMJ. For the other epileptic syndromes, the limited number of patients did not allow comparisons to be made. We noted a high frequency of consanguineous marriages in our 2 groups. The sex ratio was not statistically different, despite the existence of a slight female predominance in the EMJ group compared with the EI-CGTC group (sex ratio 0.69 and 1.27 respectively). The age of onset of epilepsy did not differ between our 2 groups. In terms of personal history, FC was more frequently observed in patients followed for EI-CGTC (20% vs 13.6%), but the difference was not significant. A family history of epilepsy was more frequent in the EMJ group, but the difference was not statistically significant. Clinical photosensitivity was more common in JME ($p = 0.01$). From a therapeutic point of view, the addition of an AE treatment was necessary mainly during AE-CGTC ($p = 0.05$), which was drug-resistant in 15% of cases. The risk of EME was not a distinguishing criterion (Table IV).In terms of electroencephalography, the standard inter-critical EEG was more frequently normal in the AE-CGTC group ($p<0.05$), since generalised inter-critical electrical abnormalities were mainly recorded during JME (0.000). The photo-paroxysmal response and electrical abnormalities triggered by HPN were also more frequently observed during JME ($p<0.05$ and $p=0.001$ respectively) (Table Ve).

Table IV: Epidemiological and clinical characteristics of patients followed for AE-CGTC and EMJ

		EI-CGTC	EMJ	P
Gender	Men	56%	40,9%	
	Woman	44%	59,1%	NS
Febrile crisis		20%	13,6%	NS
Consanguinity		40%	31,8%	NS
ATCDF for epilepsy		29%	40,9%	NS
Age of onset of epilepsy		18 +/- 10.24 years	18 +/- 7.43 years	NS
Clinical photosensitivity		2%	22,7%	0,01
EME		20%	4,5%	NS
Bi or poly therapy		42%	18,18%	0,053
Pharmaco resistance		15%	0%	

IE-CGTC: idiopathic epilepsy with isolated tonic-clonic generalised seizures; JME: juvenile myoclonic epilepsy; ATCDF: family history; SDE: status epilepticus.

Table V: EEG findings in the idiopathic epilepsy group with isolated CGTC and juvenile myoclonic epilepsy

Inter-critical EEG		EI-CGTC	EMJ	P
Normal		68,8%	28,6%	0,036
General P-PO-PP		21%	61,9%	0,000
P-PO-PP focal		13,3%	9,5%	NS
Photo-response paroxysmal		5,5%	23,8%	0,023
HPN abnormalities		4,4%	33,3%	0,001

IE-CGTC: idiopathic epilepsy with isolated tonic-clonic generalised seizures; JME: juvenile myoclonic epilepsy; P: peak; PO: peak wave; PP: poly-peak; HPN: hyperpnoea.

DISCUSSION

ELECTRO-CLINICAL SYNDROMES IN CHILDREN:

2.3.1 Epilepsy absence in children :

We included in our study subjects aged over 18 years. This inclusion criterion may explain the small number of patients followed for EAE in our series (3 patients). In most cases, the attacks disappear around the age of puberty. EAE is a generalised epilepsy of genetic origin which accounts for 1.5 to 12% of epilepsies (6).the genetic origin of this epilepsy was attested by the presence of familial cases (2 patients/3 in our series, 13 to 44% in the literature)(7-9).with regard to the mode of transmission, parental consanguinity observed in one patient in our series, and in 51% of patients in the literature(9), could indicate the importance of autosomal recessive inheritance. However, this mode of inheritance has rarely been reported for EAE and no recessive gene has been identified. In most cases, these are familial forms of complex inheritance. Contrary to the literature, where authors have concluded that EAE is more frequently observed in girls (6.9), the sex ratio was 2 in our series. However, the limited number of our patients does not allow us to draw any conclusions. A history of CF was found in only one patient in our series and in 18% of patients in 2 previous studies (8,10). The mean age of onset of epilepsy in our series (4.66 years) was comparable to that reported in previous studies (5.4 and 5.7 years) (8,9,11). Semiologically, all our adult patients presented with simple absence seizures. In contrast, in the literature, absence seizures The diagnosis of EAE in our patients was based on questioning, with a history dating back several years. It is possible that the description given by the patient or those around him was not precise enough and that his attacks were wrongly classified as simple absence attacks.In terms of electroencephalography, critical rhythmic PO discharges at 3 Hz were recorded in one patient. For the intercritical EEG, in accordance with the literature, the background rhythm was normal in all cases and paroxysmal abnormalities of the generalised PO type were recorded in one patient (12). Sensitivity to hyperpnoea, frequently found in this syndrome, was noted in only one case, and this could be explained by the administration of AE treatment before the EEG was performed. In terms of treatment, all our patients received a compound classically effective against absence seizures: VPA alone or combined with PB (13), although the latter was known to be usually ineffective (14). Under AE treatment, cure was the rule, although the occurrence of CGTC (12.8 to 60% in the literature) was a pejorative factor, and could explain the need for dual therapy in one patient in our series(11). The persistence of ECs in this patient was probably due to a poor choice of second AE (PB), making it necessary to switch to another compound.

3 THE SYNDROMES ELECTRO-CLINICAL OF ADOLESCENTS AND ADULTS :

3.1 Idiopathic generalised epilepsy with isolated tonic-clonic generalised seizures

In the literature, very few studies have looked specifically at EI-CGTC. This was the most common idiopathic epilepsy syndrome. in our series (78.7% of AEs) and in previous studies (82% of AEs in an Irish series) (15). With regard to the sex ratio, the results varied from one series to another. In our series, as well as in an Iranian series, a discrete male predominance was noted (the sex ratio was 1.27 and 1.18 respectively) (9), in contrast to a Canadian series where women were more affected than men (16). The genetic origin of this AE was suggested by the high frequency of family history of epilepsy in our series (29%), as well as in previous series (7,9,16) (10-58%). Regarding the mode of transmission, parental consanguinity, found in 40% of cases in our series and in 36-44% in the literature (7,15), indicated the possibility of recessive inheritance in this syndrome, although the pathogenesis was not yet well established. With regard to personal history, the rate of CF in our series (20%) was comparable to those reported in previous series (13 to 19%) (9,16,17). However, these attacks may be underestimated and neglected by patients. In fact, a history of CF was a risk factor for developing IE (18).The mean age of onset of epilepsy in our series and the extreme ages were comparable to those reported in an Austrian series where the mean age was 16.7 years with extremes ranging from 4 to 42 years (17). In our series, as in the literature, clinical photosensitivity was rare (2 to 3%) (17). Electrically, in this idiopathic generalised epilepsy, the typical intercritical abnormalities were generalised PO, PP or PPO. In our series, as in the literature, these abnormalities were much less frequent in IE-CGTC than in other IE (12). 13.3% of our patients had focal intercritical abnormalities. This focalisation was compatible with the diagnosis of generalised AEs in the literature (19,20), since the starting point in generalised seizures was focal with rapid bilateral involvement of cortical and subcortical areas.(21). As in our series, the frontal and temporal locations of these focal anomalies were the most frequently described (45.5% and 31.8% respectively) (19). AE-CGTC was generally associated with a good prognosis, with a favourable outcome in the majority of cases in both the literature and our series (16,17,22). However, 15% of our patients continued to have frequent attacks. Trauma related to EC was more frequent in our series than in a Canadian series (20% vs. 2%) (16). Similarly, MFE was more frequent in our series (20% vs 8.5% in the Canadian series and 4.3% in the Iranian series)(9,16).

3.2 Juvenile myoclonic epilepsy :

The incidence of JME has been estimated at 1/100,000 (23), and its prevalence among the different types of epilepsy in large cohorts has been around 5-10% (24) (5.4% in our series). Its prevalence among AEs was estimated at 17.32% in our series, which was lower than the data in the literature (26.7%)(25). A family history of epilepsy was found in 40.9% of our patients. This result varied from one ethnic group to another (23.6% to 40% in the literature) (26-28), especially as this frequency could be underestimated because patients were not obliged to give details of family cases. However, the presence of similar familial cases always argues in favour of the genetic origin of these idiopathic syndromes. In our series, the rate of consanguinity was 31.8%, which was higher than the average for all patients.of consanguineous marriages in the country (19.24%) (29). This notion suggests a autosomal recessive inheritance for JME. CF, frequently found in the questioning of patients with AE, was described by 13.6% of our patients, which is in line with the rates reported in the literature (3.2-15%) (25,26,30).The female predominance observed in our series was generally reported in most previous series (31). With regard to the age of onset of seizures, in our series, as well as in previous studies, JME began in the second decade of life, with extremes varying from 8 to 32 years of age and a peak in frequency between 12 and 18 years of age (32).The semiology of these inaugural seizures in our series was as follows: myoclonus was the first type of seizure in 59% of cases, alone or associated with CGTC in 18% of cases (33% in the literature). Isolated CGTCs inaugurated the picture in 36.36% of cases, which was close to the data in the literature (25%) (30), and absence seizures were the first type of EC in only one patient (4.5% vs 2 to 11.1% in previous series). (33). The distribution of inaugural seizures varied according to the series, but in the majority of studies they were CGTC, myoclonus, or a combination of the 2 types of seizure beginning simultaneously (30). During the course of the epilepsy, myoclonus, which is essential for diagnosis, was present in all our patients. CGTCs were also present in all our patients, as well as in the Indian series by Jayalakshmi published in 2006 (28). Absence seizures were reported in 27.2% of our patients and 31.9% of cases according to Wolf in 2015(33).1/4 of our patients had all 3 types of seizures associated, which was lower than the data from the Genton series in 2000 where all 3 types of seizures were associated in about one third of patients (35). Regarding the timing of these seizures, we found that 41% of our patients had CGTC and/or myoclonus on waking. In fact, this circadian distribution was characteristic of JME, since the majority of seizures occurred in the morning, after awakening from a nap or during sudden intermediate nocturnal awakenings (5% of our patients) (35).Clinical photosensitivity was noted in 22.7% of patients in our series. This notion was probably underestimated because it was neglected by the patient. In fact, photosensitivity was closely linked to JME, and this link has been established by Wolf and Goosses since 1986 (36), occurring in 21% of AEs and 29-42% of JMEs (33).In terms of electroencephalography, the inter-critical tracing was characterised by normal background activity (37) (all our patients) and typically rapid inter-ictal PPO and PO (54% in the literature vs 73.18% in our series) (37). These abnormalities could be generalised (61.9% of cases in our series) or predominantly frontal (9.52% in our series) (37). Focal anomalies were found in 9.52% of our patients. Their existence does not rule out the diagnosis of JME, since they can be seen in 6 to 40% of cases (37,38). The EEG may be normal (30% vs. 28.6% in our series) but this does not rule out the diagnosis of JME (39). EEG photosensitivity was reported at very variable rates (8% to 48% in the literature, 23.8% in our series). It seems that this rate depended on whether the EEG was taken before or after AE treatment (27,28). Similarly, sensitivity to hyperpnoea was frequently found (30.2% -36.7% in previous series(26,40), and33% in our series).Radiologically, all our patients had normal brain imaging.

On review of the literature, patients with JME do not appear to have structural abnormalities on conventional brain imaging (41). VPA was the most prescribed AE treatment in our series (90.9%). It was considered to be the first-line treatment for JME (42), and three other AEs were effective: VLE, topiramate and zonisamide (43). In our country, the cost and unavailability of some of these treatments limited their use. As a result, VPA remained the treatment of choice for men and women under childbearing age(44). Since 1996, the efficacy of EVL against photoparoxysmal responses and myoclonus has been proven. LMG was also effective in adult patients with JME, and better tolerated than VPA. These 2 treatments could therefore be a therapeutic alternative for women with JME of childbearing age, given the teratogenic risk of VPA (46,47,48).2 patients in our series were treated with LMG with good outcome. However, in the case of EMJ, a deleterious effect of LMG, resulting mainly in an increase in myoclonus and exceptionally in an increase in the frequency of CGTC, has been reported (47).2 publications have reported a dose-dependent effect, with an increase in myoclonus for serum LMG concentrations above 15 mg/l (49,50). In this context, it should be noted that LMG regained its full efficacy when the dosage was reduced. This explains the good response of our 2 patients. Other treatments have proved effective, such as PB (49). Only one patient in our series was treated with PB in combination with VPA, with a reduction in the frequency of attacks. In our series, as in the literature, the addition of BZDs improved the efficacy of VPA (50). Numerous AE drugs were avoided in our series, as well as in the literature (CBZ, phenytoin, oxcarbazepine, gabapentin, vigabatrin and tiagabine), given their aggravating effect on AEs, particularly JME (49). Under AE treatment, high seizure control rates have been reported in North American and European studies (70-81%) (32,51,52). almost 15%, particularly in patients with all 3 types of seizures (44). In our series, all patients were well controlled by AE treatment. In our study, only one patient presented with a seizure following discontinuation of treatment. This complication was more frequent in

Camfield's series, where 35% of patients presented with a convulsive seizure precipitated by one or more factors, essentially poor compliance with AE treatment (31).

3.3 Epilepsy absence juvenile

EAJ is an uncommon epileptic syndrome (1.57% of AEs in our series, 0.84% to 11.1% in the literature), but it should be borne in mind that it may be unrecognised and therefore underestimated (15,53). The age of onset of EC ranged from 8 to 17 years, with a peak at 10-12 years (9,12,54), but late onset in adulthood was also reported in 2 of our patients (19 and 20 years) (9,54). family history of EC was not found in our two patients, contrary to the literature where it has been frequently noted (40 to 50%) (8,9,54). This type of EC may not be recognised by family members. Parental consanguinity was noted in one of the 2 patients in our series. However, in a population from Saudi Arabia (55), consanguinity was found in only one of 14 families with EAJ. This finding was not in favour of recessive inheritance. CF, present in only one patient in our series, was rarely reported in the literature(8). In our series, absence seizures were typically simple in one patient and typically complex in the second. The type of absence seizures was not specified in the various series in the literature (9,54,55), and the frequency of these seizures was lower than that described in EAE (54). However, in EAJ, myoclonus was more frequent than in EAE. frequently found (no patients in our study), and CGTCs may even precede absence seizures (12,54). On EEG, the background rhythm was normal in our 2 patients and in the series reported in the literature. Typical intercritical abnormalities were generalised PO discharges, but an anterior predominance of abnormalities, found in our 2 patients, has been described in some series (56). In terms of treatment, one patient was treated with VPA combined with a BZD (13), and the other patient with LEV. Drug resistance is more frequent in cases where absence seizures are associated with CGTCs, as was the case in our second patient. Epilepsy has been complicated by an MEE in 6% of cases in the literature(9) and in one patient in our study.

4 ANALYSIS STATISTICS:

We tried to find distinctive features between EI-CGTC and EMJ. The age of onset did not differ between our 2 groups, since these were 2 electroclinical syndromes of adolescents and adults. The demographic and clinical characteristics of the patients were sometimes different, but this difference was not always statistically significant.Among the clinical characteristics noted in our work were the high frequency of consanguinity and family history of epilepsy in our two groups. In fact, the non-significant difference in the results for these 2 parameters, also observed in the literature (10), could be explained by the presumed genetic basis of all idiopathic epileptic syndromes. In our study, as well as in the literature, a female predominance was observed in JME (9), except that in our study, this result was not statistically significant, probably due to the small number of our patients. As regards personal history of CF, in accordance with the literature, we noted a higher frequency of group, in contrast to clinical photosensitivity, which was more frequent in the JME group.From an electrical point of view, the EEG provided us with additional arguments, apart from the clinical elements, in the positive diagnosis of AR. However, it can sometimes be non-contributory and even misleading (59). It was normal in 11-45% of cases, depending on the series (9,57). This frequency varied according to the epileptic syndrome. In our series, normal intercritical EEGs were more common in patients with EI-CGTC, and the difference was significant. In previous studies (9,57), JME w a s   m o r e   associated with normal recordings. In fact, it seems that the EEG depends on whether or not AE treatment is being taken, and since the majority of patients in the EI-CGTC group were initially followed up in other health structures and were referred to us secondarily, the EEG was recorded in patients who had been treated for several years, which could explain the absence of electrical abnormalities in 68.8% of our patients. The second limitation of the EEG was the lack of specificity of the inter-critical abnormalities observed. Indeed, in all generalised AE syndromes, generalised P, PP and PO could be recorded (9). In our study, these abnormalities were mainly encountered during JME, with a significant difference. On the other hand, during these generalised syndromes, focal electrical abnormalities could be recorded (9). In accordance with the data in the literature (9,57), the photo-paroxysmal response and paroxysmal abnormalities triggered by HPN were more frequently observed in the group of patients with JME, and the difference was significant in our study.

5 THE LIMITATIONS OF OUR STUDY :

-EEG was performed in only 116 of the 127 patients in our series. In fact, for patients referred to us from in whom the epilepsy was well controlled, an EEG was not requested, as it would most likely be normal.

CONCLUSION

AEs are a group of heterogeneous epileptic syndromes, with specific clinico-electrical and evolutionary characteristics. The prevalence of AEs varied widely between studies, probably due to ethnic variations and methodological differences.We retained 127 cases of AE (3 EAE, 100 EI-CGTC, 22 EMJ and 2 EAJ). The frequency of AEs was 31.2% of all patients with epilepsy. This figure was lower than expected according to the literature. This could be explained by a recruitment bias; in fact, we only included patients aged over 18 in our study. Given that AEs are age-dependent syndromes, occurring most often in childhood and adolescence, limiting the study to the adult population will result in a lower percentage of AEs. We noted a high frequency of consanguinity in our series, suggesting autosomal recessive inheritance for AR. This mode of inheritance was rarely described in the literature.The clinical and electrical characteristics of the various syndromes diagnosed in our series were broadly consistent with the literature. The main distinguishing clinical features between CGTC-IE and JME were the sex ratio, with a female predominance, clinical photosensitivity and pharmaco-sensitivity, which were more frequent in JME. In terms of electroencephalography, more than half of our patients had a normal EEG. The absence of inter-critical abnormalities was more frequently observed in our EI-CGTC patients. On the other hand, generalised inter-critical abnormalities, photo-paroxysmal response and paroxysmal abnormalities triggered by HPN were more frequently observed in the group of patients with JME. Sodium valproate, the most widely prescribed drug in our series, was effective in the various AE syndromes, since EC was controlled in the majority of cases (all our patients followed for JME and 85% of patients with AE-CGTC). As a result, epilepsy did not impair the quality of life of our patients and did not limit their schooling or their integration into working life.At the end of our study, we emphasise the importance of meticulous questioning to look for the notion of myoclonus or absence seizures, which are often neglected by patients and their families, and whose presence has important therapeutic implications. We also found that focal inter-critical EEG abnormalities were described during generalised AEs, which may be a source of confusion and misdiagnosis as focal epilepsy, with prescription of potentially aggravating AEs. AEs could begin at a late age. The diagnosis would then be made after ruling out a cerebral lesion that could explain the clinico-electrical picture, since symptomatic epilepsies are most common in adults and elderly subjects. Better knowledge of the main clinico-electrical and evolutionary characteristics of the various AR syndromes could therefore improve the management of patients with epilepsy in our country and better guide subsequent epidemiological and genetic studies.

SUMMARY

INTRODUCTION

Idiopathic epilepsy (IE) accounts for 20% of epilepsies, but less than 1% of research into this disease. This imbalance reflects a lack of awareness of the diagnostic difficulties, particularly in cases of late onset or atypical signs.
PATIENTS AND METHOD

We conducted a retrospective study including adults followed for AE. We identified the distinctive clinical and paraclinical criteria of the different syndromes in adults.
RESULTS :

EI-CGTC was the most frequent epileptic syndrome (78.7%) followed by JME (17.32%). A family history of epilepsy and clinical photosensitivity were more common in JME (p=0.01). Electroencephalographic findings showed that generalised intercritical abnormalities, photoparoxysmal response and HPN-triggered electrical abnormalities were most common in JME (p=0.000, p<0.05 and 0.001 respectively). Focal abnormalities were recorded during these 2 syndromes.
CONCLUSIONS :

Knowledge of the characteristics of AR syndromes could improve patient management and better guide subsequent epidemiological and genetic studies.

BIBLIOGRAPHY

1. Fisher RS, Acevedo C, Arzimanoglou A, Bogacz A, Cross JH, Elger CE, et al. ILAE official report: a practical clinical definition of epilepsy. Epilepsia. Apr 2014;55(4):475-82.

2. Edouard Hirsch, Jacqueline French, Ingrid E. Scheffer, Alicia Bogacz, Taoufik Alsaadi,| Michael R. Sperlin, Fatema Abda, | Sameer M, Zuberi et al. Sperlin, Fatema Abda, Sameer M, Zuberi et al. ILAE definition of the Idiopathic Generalized Epilepsy Syndromes: Position statement by the ILAE Task Force on Nosology and Definitions. Epilepsia 2022;63:1475-1499.

3. Scheffer IE, Berkovic S, Capovilla G, Connolly MB, French J, Guilhoto L, et al. ILAE classification of the epilepsies: Position paper of the ILAE Commission for Classification and Terminology. Epilepsia. Apr 2017;58(4):512-21.

4. Hauser WA. Recent developments in the epidemiology of epilepsy. Acta Neurol Scand Suppl. 1995;162:17-21.

5. Reichsoellner J, Larch J, Unterberger I, Dobesberger J, Kuchukhidze G, Luef G, et al. Idiopathic generalised epilepsy of late onset: a separate nosological entity? J Neurol Neurosurg Psychiatry. Nov 2010;81(11):1218-22.

6. Asadi-Pooya AA, Emami M, Nikseresht A. Early-onset versus typical childhood absence epilepsy; clinical and electrographic characteristics. Seizure. 1 May 2012;21(4):273-5.

7. Ndiaye M, Sarr MM, Mapouré Y, Sène-Diouf F, Touré K, Sow AD, et al [Epilepsy in a cohort of Senegalese children]. Rev Neurol (Paris). Feb 2008;164(2):162-8.

8. Sadleir LG, Scheffer IE, Smith S, Connolly MB, Farrell K. Automatisms in absence seizures in children with idiopathic generalized epilepsy. Arch Neurol. June 2009;66(6):729-34.

9. Asadi-Pooya AA, Emami M, Sperling MR. A clinical study of syndromes of idiopathic (genetic) generalized epilepsy. J Neurol Sci. 15 Jan 2013;324(1):113-7.

10. Ma X, Zhang Y, Yang Z, Liu X, Sun H, Qin J, et al. Childhood absence epilepsy: Elctroclinical features and diagnostic criteria. Brain Dev. Feb 2011;33(2):114-9.

11. Callenbach PMC, Bouma PAD, Geerts AT, Arts WFM, Stroink H, Peeters EAJ, et al. Long-term outcome of childhood absence epilepsy: Dutch Study of Epilepsy in Childhood. Epilepsy Res. Feb 2009;83(2-3):249-56.

12. Seneviratne U, Cook MJ, D'Souza WJ. Electroencephalography in the Diagnosis of Genetic Generalized Epilepsy Syndromes. Front Neurol. 2017;8:499.

13. Glauser TA, Cnaan A, Shinnar S, Hirtz DG, Dlugos D, Masur D, et al. Ethosuximide, valproic acid, and lamotrigine in childhood absence epilepsy: initial monotherapy outcomes at 12 months. Epilepsia. Jan 2013;54(1):141-55.

14. Sazgar M, Bourgeois BFD. Aggravation of epilepsy by antiepileptic drugs. Pediatr Neurol. Oct 2005;33(4):227-34.

15. Mullins GM, O'Sullivan SS, Neligan A, McCarthy A, McNamara B, Galvin RJ, et al. A study of idiopathic generalised epilepsy in an Irish population. Seizure. 1 Apr 2007;16(3):204-10.

16. Camfield P, Camfield C. Idiopathic generalized epilepsy with generalized tonic-clonic seizures (IGE-GTC): a population-based cohort with >20 year

follow up for medical and social outcome. Epilepsy Behav EB. May 2010;18(1-2):61-3.

17. Unterberger I, Trinka E, Luef G, Bauer G. Idiopathic generalized epilepsies with pure grand mal: clinical data and genetics. Epilepsy Res. Apr 2001;44(1):19-25.

18. Li M, Heng X, Tao R, Liu J, Zhang L, Sun X, et al. A genetic epidemiological survey of idiopathic epilepsy in the Chinese Han population. Epilepsy Res. Feb 2012;98(2-3):199-205.

19. Esmail EH, Nawito AM, Labib DM, Basheer MA. Focal interictal epileptiform discharges in idiopathic generalized epilepsy. Neurol Sci Off J Ital Neurol Soc Ital Soc Clin Neurophysiol. jul 2016;37(7):1071-7.

20. Seneviratne U, Cook M, D'Souza W. Focal abnormalities in idiopathic generalized epilepsy: a critical review of the literature. Epilepsia. August 2014;55(8):1157-69.

21. Berg AT, Berkovic SF, Brodie MJ, Buchhalter J, Cross JH, van Emde Boas W, et al. Revised terminology and concepts for organization of seizures and epilepsies: report of the ILAE Commission on Classification and Terminology, 2005-2009. Epilepsia. Apr 2010;51(4):676-85.

22. Michel VHN, Sebban C, Debray-Meignan S, Ourabah Z, Rousseau-Lavallard MC, Piette F, et al. Electroclinical features of idiopathic generalized epilepsies in the elderly: a geriatric hospital-based study. Seizure. May 2011;20(4):292-8.

23. Jallon P, Latour P. Epidemiology of idiopathic generalized epilepsies. Epilepsia. 2005;46 Suppl 9:10-4.

24. Syvertsen MR, Thuve S, Stordrange BS, Brodtkorb E. Clinical heterogeneity

of juvenile myoclonic epilepsy: follow-up after an interval of more than 20 years. Seizure. May 2014;23(5):344-8.

25. Martínez-Juárez IE, Alonso ME, Medina MT, Durón RM, Bailey JN, López-Ruiz M, et al. Juvenile myoclonic epilepsy subsyndromes: family studies and long-term follow-up. Brain. 1 May 2006;129(5):1269-80.

26. Canevini MP, Mai R, Di Marco C, Bertin C, Minotti L, Pontrelli V, et al. Juvenile myoclonic epilepsy of Janz: clinical observations in 60 patients. Seizure. 1 Dec 1992;1(4):291-8.

27. Murthy JM, Rao CM, Meena AK. Clinical observations of juvenile myoclonic epilepsy in 131 patients: a study in South India. Seizure. Feb 1998;7(1):43-7.

28. Jayalakshmi SS, Mohandas S, Sailaja S, Borgohain R. Clinical and electroencephalographic study of first-degree relatives and probands with juvenile myoclonic epilepsy. Seizure. Apr 2006;15(3):177-83.

29. BenMRad.pdf [Internet]. [cited 14 Dec 2017]. Available from: http://www.didac.ehu.es/antropo/12/12-6/BenMRad.pdf

30. Genton P, Thomas P, Kasteleijn-Nolst Trenité DGA, Medina MT, Salas-Puig J. Clinical aspects of juvenile myoclonic epilepsy. Epilepsy Behav EB. Jul 2013;28 Suppl 1:S8-14.

31. Camfield CS, Camfield PR. Juvenile myoclonic epilepsy 25 years after seizure onset: a population-based study. Neurology. 29 Sep 2009;73(13):1041-5.

32. Panayiotopoulos CP, Obeid T, Tahan AR. Juvenile myoclonic epilepsy: a 5-year prospective study. Epilepsia. Apr 1994;35(2):285-96.

33. Wolf P, Yacubian EMT, Avanzini G, Sander T, Schmitz B, Wandschneider

B, et al. Juvenile myoclonic epilepsy: A system disorder of the brain. Epilepsy Res. August 2015;114:2-12.

34. Manford M. Juvenile Myoclonic Epilepsy: the Janz Syndrome. J Neurol Neurosurg Psychiatry. 1 Dec 2000;69(6):838-838.

35. Zarowski M, Loddenkemper T, Vendrame M, Alexopoulos AV, Wyllie E, Kothare SV. Circadian distribution and sleep/wake patterns of generalized seizures in children. Epilepsia. June 2011;52(6):1076-83.

36. Wolf P, Goosses R. Relation of photosensitivity to epileptic syndromes. J Neurol Neurosurg Psychiatry. Dec 1986;49(12):1386-91.

37. Serafini A, Rubboli G, Gigli GL, Koutroumanidis M, Gelisse P. Neurophysiology of juvenile myoclonic epilepsy. Epilepsy Behav EB. Jul 2013;28 Suppl 1:S30-39.

38. Aliberti V, Grünewald RA, Panayiotopoulos CP, Chroni E. Focal electroencephalographic abnormalities in juvenile myoclonic epilepsy. Epilepsia. Apr 1994;35(2):297-301.

39. Shahnaz null, Sher K, Abdul Sattar R. Clinical and EEG characteristics of Juvenile Myoclonic Epilepsy. Pak J Med Sci. Jan 2014;30(1):12-5.

40. Montalenti E, Imperiale D, Rovera A, Bergamasco B, Benna P. Clinical features, EEG findings and diagnostic pitfalls in juvenile myoclonic epilepsy: a series of 63 patients. J Neurol Sci. 15 Feb 2001;184(1):65-70.

41. Lin K, Jackowski AP, Carrete H, de Araújo Filho GM, Silva HH, Guaranha MSB, et al. Voxel-based morphometry evaluation of patients with photosensitive juvenile myoclonic epilepsy. Epilepsy Res. Oct 2009;86(2-3):138-45.

42. Chowdhury A, Brodie MJ. Pharmacological outcomes in juvenile myoclonic epilepsy: Support for sodium valproate. Epilepsy Res. Jan 2016;119:62-6.

43. Asadi-Pooya AA, Hashemzehi Z, Emami M. Predictors of seizure control in patients with juvenile myoclonic epilepsy (JME). Seizure. nov 2014;23(10):889-91.

44. Auvin S. Treatment of myoclonic seizures in patients with juvenile myoclonic epilepsy. Neuropsychiatr Dis Treat. Dec 2007;3(6):729-34.

45. Nicolson A, Marson AG. When the first antiepileptic drug fails in a patient with juvenile myoclonic epilepsy. Pract Neurol. August 2010;10(4):208-18.

46. Geddes JR, Calabrese JR, Goodwin GM. Lamotrigine for treatment of bipolar depression: independent meta-analysis and meta-regression of individual patient data from five randomised trials. Br J Psychiatry J Ment Sci. Jan 2009;194(1):4-9.

47. Crespel A, Genton P, Berramdane M, Coubes P, Monicard C, Baldy-Moulinier M, et al. Lamotrigine associated with exacerbation or de novo myoclonus in idiopathic generalized epilepsies. Neurology. 13 Sept 2005;65(5):762-4.

48. Janszky J, Rásonyi G, Halász P, Olajos S, Perényi J, Szûcs A, et al. Disabling erratic myoclonus during lamotrigine therapy with high serum level--report of two cases. Clin Neuropharmacol. Apr 2000;23(2):86-9.

49. Crespel A, Gelisse P, Reed RC, Ferlazzo E, Jerney J, Schmitz B, et al. Management of juvenile myoclonic epilepsy. Epilepsy Behav EB. Jul 2013;28 Suppl 1:S81-86.

50. Obeid T, Panayiotopoulos CP. Clonazepam in juvenile myoclonic epilepsy. Epilepsia. Oct 1989;30(5):603-6.

51. Jayalakshmi S, Vooturi S, Bana AK, Sailaja S, Somayajula S, Mohandas S. Factors associated with lack of response to valproic acid monotherapy in juvenile myoclonic epilepsy. Seizure. August 2014;23(7):527-32.

52. Fernando-Dongas MC, Radtke RA, VanLandingham KE, Husain AM. Characteristics of valproic acid resistant juvenile myoclonic epilepsy. Seizure. Sept 2000;9(6):385-8.

53. Mahoney K, Buckley D, Alam M, Penney S, Young TL, Parfrey P, et al. High incidence of pediatric idiopathic epilepsy is associated with familial and autosomal dominant disease in Eastern Newfoundland. Epilepsy Res. Feb 2012;98(2-3):140-7.

54. Aiguabella Macau M, Falip Centellas M, Veciana de Las Heras M, Climent Perín MA, Miró Lladó J, Moreno Gómez I, et al. Long term prognosis of juvenile absence epilepsy. Neurol Barc Spain. May 2011;26(4):193-9.

55. Obeid T. Clinical and genetic aspects of juvenile absence epilepsy. J Neurol. July 1994;241(8):487-91.

56. Gelisse P, Serafini A, Velizarova R, Genton P, Crespel A. Temporal intermittent δ activity: a marker of juvenile absence epilepsy? Seizure. Jan 2011;20(1):38-41.

57. Betting LE, Mory SB, Lopes-Cendes I, Li LM, Guerreiro MM, Guerreiro CAM, et al. EEG features in idiopathic generalized epilepsy: clues to diagnosis. Epilepsia. March 2006;47(3):523-8.

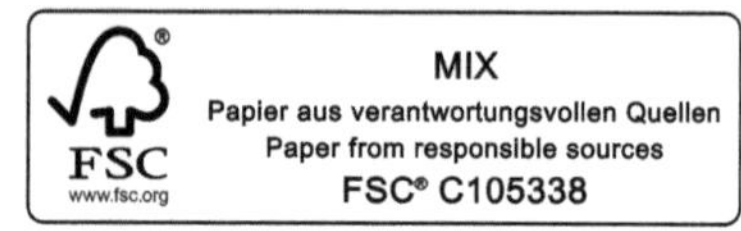

Printed by Books on Demand GmbH, Norderstedt / Germany